Sameh Belgacem

Leishmaniasis in Tunisia

Sameh Belgacem

Leishmaniasis in Tunisia

Leishmaniasis in Tunisia: Epidemiology, Clinical Presentations and Diagnostic Strategies

ScienciaScripts

Imprint
Any brand names and product names mentioned in this book are subject to trademark, brand or patent protection and are trademarks or registered trademarks of their respective holders. The use of brand names, product names, common names, trade names, product descriptions etc. even without a particular marking in this work is in no way to be construed to mean that such names may be regarded as unrestricted in respect of trademark and brand protection legislation and could thus be used by anyone.

Cover image: www.ingimage.com

This book is a translation from the original published under ISBN 978-620-6-72808-5.

Publisher:
Sciencia Scripts
is a trademark of
Dodo Books Indian Ocean Ltd. and OmniScriptum S.R.L publishing group

120 High Road, East Finchley, London, N2 9ED, United Kingdom
Str. Armeneasca 28/1, office 1, Chisinau MD-2012, Republic of Moldova, Europe
Managing Directors: Ieva Konstantinova, Victoria Ursu
info@omniscriptum.com

Printed at: see last page
ISBN: 978-620-6-76456-4

CONTENTS

LIST OF ABBREVIATIONS

LC: cutaneous leishmaniasis

LV visceral leishmaniasis

WHO: World Health Organization

PCR: Polymerase Chain Reaction

RFLP: Restriction Fragments Length Polymorphisms

PFGE: Pulsed Field Gel Electrophoresis

SSCP: Single Strand Conformational Polymorphism

LCL: Localized cutaneous leishmaniasis

LCD: Diffuse cutaneous leishmaniasis

LCZ: Zoonotic cutaneous leishmaniasis

LCS: Sporadic cutaneous leishmaniasis

INTRODUCTION

Leishmaniasis is a group of parasitic diseases caused by a flagellate protozoan belonging to the genus *Leishmania*. They can affect several mammalian species, including man. They are transmitted by an insect vector of the genus *Phlebotomus* in the Old World and *Lutzomyia* in the New World.

The clinical expression of this parasitosis depends on the *Leishmania* species involved and the host's immune response. It includes visceral, cutaneous and mucocutaneous forms.

Leishmaniasis is a worldwide public health problem. According to World Health Organization (WHO) figures, an estimated 370 million people are exposed to the disease. The number of new cases diagnosed annually is estimated at 0.5 million for the visceral form and around one million for the cutaneous form.

In recent years, several molecular methods have been developed for the detection and identification of *Leishmania*. Lack of standardization, homogenization and validation are the main drawbacks of these tools. The WHO "Tropical Diseases Research" TDR technical report on research priorities for leishmaniasis highlighted the need to standardize and validate molecular tests.

1. . Epidemiology

The epidemiological study of leishmaniasis involves analyzing the elements of the parasite cycle, namely the parasite, the vector and the reservoir.

1.1. Pathogen

1.1.1. Taxonomic position

Leishmania parasites belong to (1) :
Kingdom: *Protista*
Class: *Kinetoplastea*
Subclass: *Metakinetoplastina*
Order: *Trypanosomatida*
Family: *Trypanosomatidae*
Subfamily: *Leishmaniinae*
Genre: *Leishmania*

Some 30 species of this genus have been recorded, over two-thirds of which are pathogenic to humans. They are grouped into two subgenera according to their development around the pylorus of the vector intestine: subgenus *Leishmania* has supra-pyloric development and subgenus *Viannia* has peri-pyloric development(2,3).

Since 1981, isoenzyme electrophoresis, recognized by the WHO, has been the reference technique for identifying *Leishmania* strains, but biology techniques such as PCR-sequencing (Polymerase Chain Reaction), RFLP (Restriction Fragments Length Polymorphisms), PFGE (Pulsed Field Gel Electrophoresis) and SSCP (Single Strand Conformational Polymorphism)(1,4,5) are increasingly being used.

1.1.2. Morphology

The morphological characteristics of all *Leishmania* species are similar. This parasite can take two evolutionary forms: the amastigote and the promastigote.

Amastigote stage

The amastigote is 2-5 ^m in size and ovoid in shape. Its identifying features are the nucleus and the kinetoplast. This form is intracellular, and is found in mononuclear phagocytic cells of vertebrate hosts. It multiplies by binary fission (6) (Figure 1).

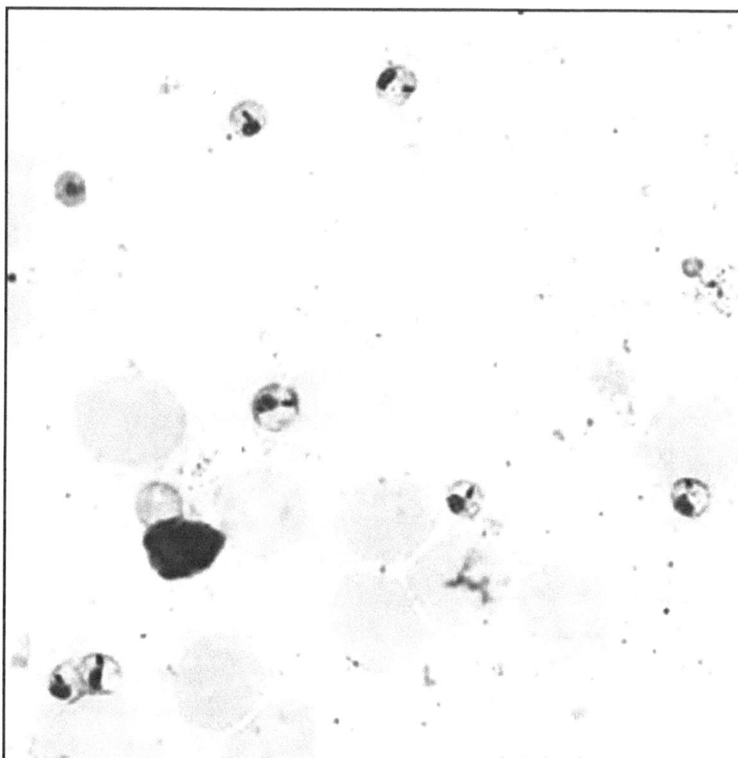

Figure 1: *Leishmania* amastigote stage (7)

Promastigote stage

It has an elongated shape, about 10 to 25 ^m long. It has an approximately central nucleus and an anterior kinetoplast from which the flagellum escapes. This stage is observed in the digestive tract of the sandfly and in *in vitro* culture media (8) (Figure 2).

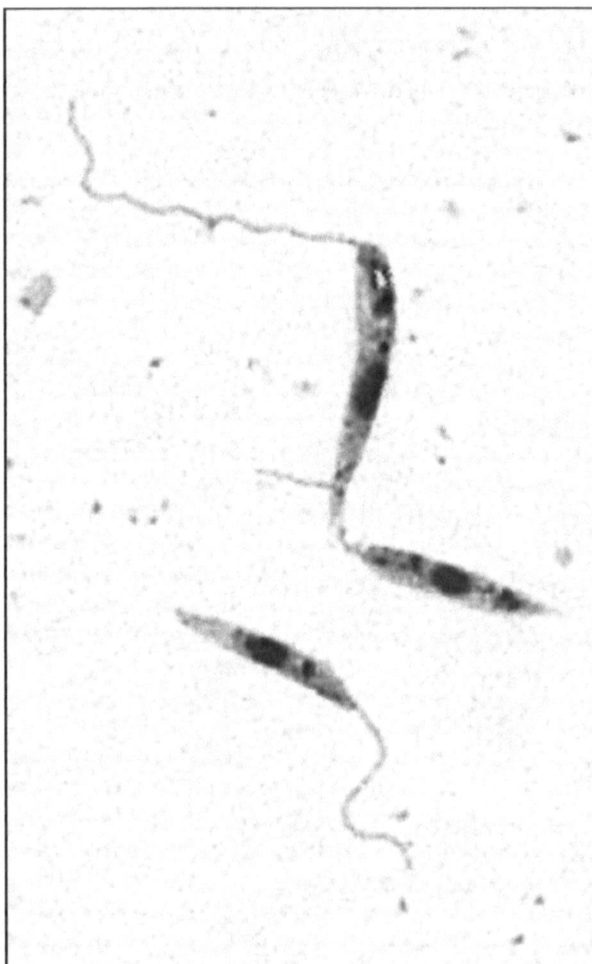

Figure 2: *Leishmania* promastigote stage (9)

1.2. Vector

The sandfly is an important link in the chain of transmission of leishmaniasis. To date, over 800 species are thought to exist in different parts of the world. They are grouped in the suborder *Nematocera* of the order *Diptera,* family *Psychodidae,* subfamily *Phlebotominae.* This subfamily is subdivided into six genera: three from the Old World (*Phlebotomus*, *Sergentomyia* and *Chinius*) and three from the New World (*Lutzomyia*, *Brumptomyia* and *Warileya*)(10).

Sandflies are mainly found in warmer regions. They undergo a complete metamorphosis through their developmental stages (egg, larva, nymph and adult). Unlike mosquitoes, the immature stages do not require stagnant water to complete their development, although they do need heat and humidity (11).

Adults are small, rarely exceeding 3.5 mm in length. They are covered with dense hairs. They have a humped appearance. At rest, they hold their wings in a characteristic "V" shape. Their color ranges from whitish to blackish. Their legs are very long and slender. The male has a highly developed genital framework. The male's genital armature, spermathecae and buccal armature are highly variable in morphology. As a result, they are the most widely used in species identification and classification (11) (figure 3). (Depaquit and Léger, 2017).

Only female sandflies need a blood meal to complete the maturation of their eggs. These insects are crepuscular and nocturnal. During the day, they hide in secluded, quiet, dark and relatively damp places (burrows, stables, hutches, niches and even houses). It is in these resting places that the eggs are laid. Their flight distance is generally very short (around 300 m), so their activity is generally limited to the vicinity of larval breeding sites. Their bites are very painful. Unlike mosquitoes, their attack on the host is silent. The lifespan of adults depends on temperature and humidity (11) (Depaquit and Léger, 2017).

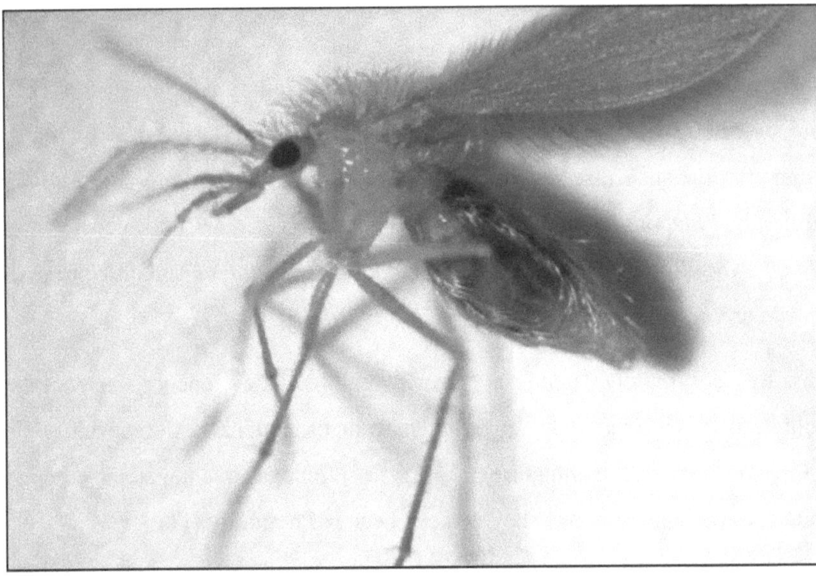

Figure 3: Photo of female sandfly gorged with blood (Laboratoire de parasitologie-Mycologie Médicale et Moléculaire, Faculté de Pharmacie de Monastir).

1.3. Tank

The mere presence of an infestation in a given mammalian species, even when it affects a large number of individuals, does not necessarily mean that the species in question is a reservoir host. For a host to be officially recognized as a reservoir, the following criteria must be taken into account (12) :

- A reservoir host must be of sufficient size and longevity to provide sandflies with an abundant food source.
- Intense contact between host and sandfly is essential. This is why many Old World reservoir hosts are gregarious animals that provide suitable habitats (e.g. burrows) for vector sandflies. A sandfly that has bitten a reservoir host therefore has a good chance of subsequently biting another, and thus transmitting the parasite within the reservoir host population.

• The proportion of individuals infested during their lifetime must be high,

• Infestation in the reservoir host must last long enough, and be sufficiently non-pathogenic, for the parasites to survive a season when there is no transmission.

• Parasites must be present in the skin or blood in sufficient numbers to pass into the sandfly's body.

Several mammal species have been identified as reservoir hosts for *Leishmania*, including dogs, rodents and damans....

Man is directly involved as the main reservoir host for visceral leishmaniasis caused by *L. donovani* and cutaneous leishmaniasis caused by *L. tropica*(12).

1.4 Transmission cycle

The *Leishmania* parasite has a tenene cycle that requires two hosts, a female sandfly and a mammal. During its blood meal, the infected female sandfly injects the infecting stage (promastigotes) into the vertebrate host through its proboscis. Promastigotes reaching the puncture site are phagocytosed by mononuclear phagocytic cells. Within these cells, promastigotes transform into amastigote stages, which multiply by binary division . Several factors, including the species of *Leishmania* involved and the host's immune response, determine whether infection becomes symptomatic or remains asymptomatic, and whether the result is cutaneous or visceral leishmaniasis.

During a blood meal in a parasitized mammal, sandflies become infected by ingesting amastigotes. Back in the vector's digestive tract, the amastigotes again differentiate into promastigotes. At first, they are in the pro-cyclic stage, actively dividing. After four days, they differentiate into nectomonads, which attach to the microvilli of midgut epithelial cells via a flagellum. From day 7, the parasites migrate to the anterior part of the intestine. Here, they transform into leptomonads, then into metacyclic promastigotes. Metacyclic promastigotes represent the infectious form for mammals. They are thinner, unable to divide and highly mobile thanks to a long flagellum (13) (figure 4).

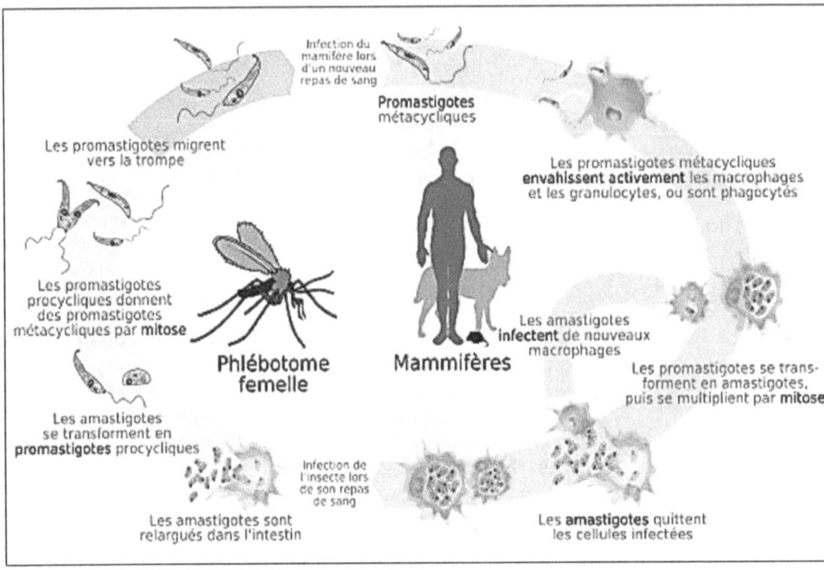

Figure 4: transmission cycle of leishmaniasis(14)

1.5. Geographical distribution

Widespread across the globe, leishmaniasis is found in the tropical and subtropical zones of 88 countries on all five continents. According to the latest WHO estimates, there are between 700,000 and 1 million new cases each year, with an incidence of between 50,000 and 90,000 new cases of visceral leishmaniasis, and between 600,000 and 1 million new cases of cutaneous leishmaniasis. Worldwide mortality attributable to this parasitosis is estimated at between 20,000 and 30,000 deaths (15).

The various forms, whether visceral, cutaneous or mucocutaneous, have territories whose delimitation depends on intrinsic factors linked to the parasite species, vector sandflies and reservoir mammals, but also on extrinsic, environmental factors.

The geographical distribution of leishmaniasis can be summarized as follows (15):

- Visceral leishmaniasis: Indian, Mediterranean, Chinese, American and African foci. In 2015, over 90% of cases notified to WHO occurred in 7 countries: Brazil, Ethiopia, India, Kenya, Somalia, Sudan and South Sudan.

-Cutaneous leishmaniasis: Mediterranean, American, African foci. In 2015, more than two-thirds of cases were recorded in the following 6 countries: Afghanistan, Algeria, Brazil, Colombia, the Syrian Arab Republic and the Islamic Republic of Iran.

-Mucocutaneous leishmaniasis: concentrated in South American countries Over 90% of cases of mucocutaneous leishmaniasis occur in Brazil, the Plurinational State of Bolivia and Peru.

1.6. Factors influencing epidemiology

The different forms of leishmaniasis - visceral, cutaneous or mucocutaneous - have territories whose delimitation depends on extrinsic, environmental factors.

1.6.1. Socio-economic factors

Socio-economic factors have a certain impact on the incidence of leishmaniasis. Poor housing conditions and peri-domestic hygiene (e.g. lack of waste management, open sewers) can increase the number of breeding and resting places for sandflies, as well as their access to humans. In addition, poor nutritional status due to poor diet increases the likelihood of visceral leishmanial infestation progressing to clinical disease (12).

1.6.2. Population displacement

Population movements have a major impact on the risk of acquiring leishmaniasis: epidemics of both visceral and cutaneous leishmaniasis are often linked to the penetration of non-immunized people into zoonotic foci of leishmaniasis, such as the extension of suburbs into the natural habitats of the vector and reservoir hosts, population migrations during wars or periods of drought (12).

1.6.3. Ecological transformations

Ecological transformations due to human activity are also likely to influence the incidence of leishmaniasis, such as urbanization, the irruption of farms, deforestation and the destruction of natural biotopes. These activities have a major impact on the ecology of vectors and reservoir hosts (12).

1.6.4. Climate change

Leishmaniasis is a disease influenced by climatic changes (rainfall, temperature and humidity), which have powerful effects on the ecology of vectors and reservoir hosts, modifying their distribution and influencing their survival and population size. The epidemiology of leishmaniasis is mainly characterized by marked seasonal and interannual fluctuations. These fluctuations are caused by climatic factors, the dynamics of vector and reservoir host populations, and the behaviour and movements of human populations (12,16).

1.6.5. Concomitant H.I.V. infection

According to the World Health Organization (WHO), around 35 million people worldwide are living with HIV. Immunosuppression has the potential to reactivate latent *Leishmania* infection in asymptomatic HIV-positive patients (17,18).

Recently, leishmaniasis has emerged as an opportunistic disease in HIV patients living in endemic areas. Furthermore, it has been noted that the risk of clinical VL in HIV patients has increased from 100 to 1,000). The proportion of patients with HIV-associated VL rose from 18.5% in 199899 to 40% in 2006(19-21).

2. Clinical picture

Clinical manifestations of leishmaniasis vary according to the characteristics of the parasite and the host's immune response. The clinical forms of this parasitosis are cutaneous (localized or diffuse), mucocutaneous and visceral.

2.1. Cutaneous leishmaniasis (LC)

2.1.1. Localized cutaneous leishmaniasis (LCL)

It occurs in areas of the body exposed to insect bites. The incubation period is 1 to 4 weeks, but can last several years. The "classic" lesion begins as an erythematous papule at the site of the bite, which develops into a vesicle and later a pustule. When the pustule ruptures, a rounded ulcer with nodular margins is formed, covered by an adherent crust. This ulcer can last from 3 months to several years. In the absence of bacterial superinfection, the lesion remains painless. In the absence of treatment, LCL may heal spontaneously in a few months, leaving an unsightly scar with altered pigmentation Old World cutaneous leishmaniasis is caused by five species of leishmania: *L. infantum, L. tropica, L. major, L. aethiopica and L. donovani* (22). (Figure 5)

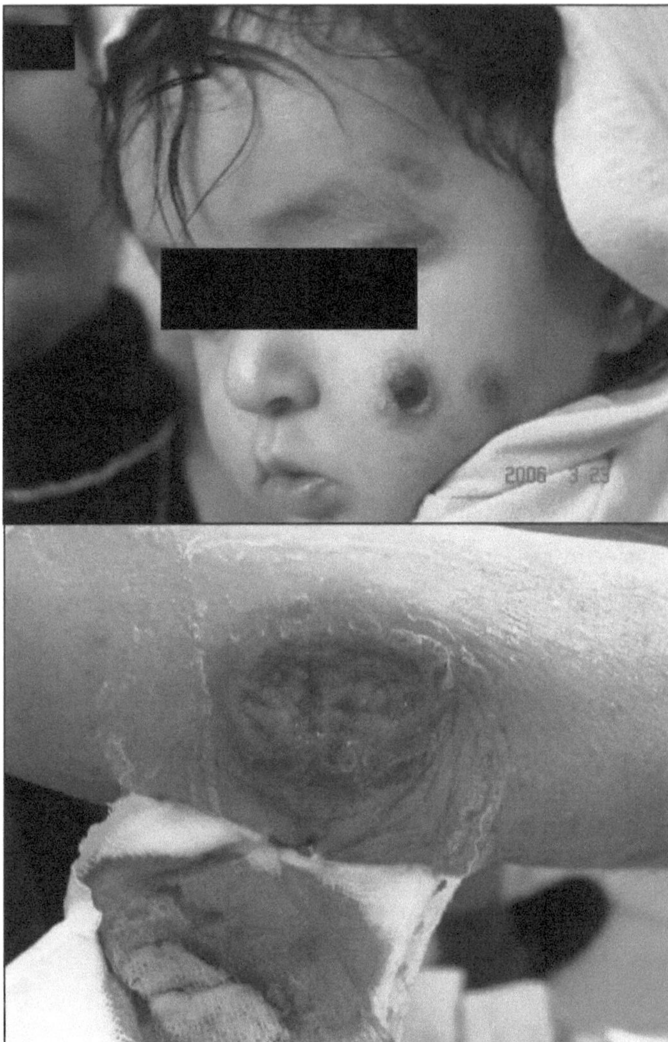

Figure 5: examples of localized cutaneous leishmaniasis lesions (Parasitology laboratory, CHU Monastir)

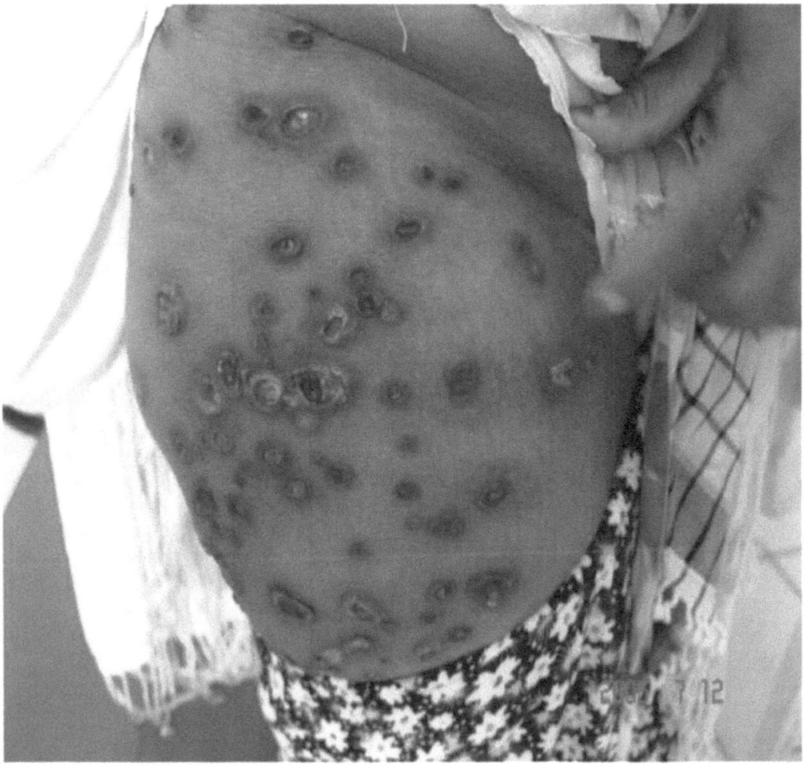

Figure 6: Multiple lesions of cutaneous leishmaniasis on the thigh (Laboratoire de Parasitologie CHU Monastir).

2.1.2. Diffuse cutaneous leishmaniasis (LCD)

This form is characterized by a lack of cellular immune response to parasite antigens. This allows the parasite to spread via tissue, lymphatic and blood routes, leading to the development of lesions throughout most of the body, sometimes associated with mucosal involvement. This form is found in Central America, Amazonian Brazil, Venezuela, Ethiopia and Kenya. It can be caused by *L. aethiopica, L. mexicana* and *L. amazonensis*. It is generally accompanied by adenopathy, altered general condition and fever. Unlike LCL, LCD does not resolve spontaneously and is very difficult to treat (22).

2.2. Mucocutaneous leishmaniasis

In South America, it has been noted that in 1 to 10% of patients, the LCL form can evolve into mucocutaneous leishmaniasis after 5 years of recovery. The species causing this form belong to the *L. braziliensis* complex, which includes *L. braziliensis*, *L. guyanensis* and *L. panamensis*. It causes invasion and destruction of the nasopharyngeal mucosa. It almost never heals spontaneously (22) (Figure 6).

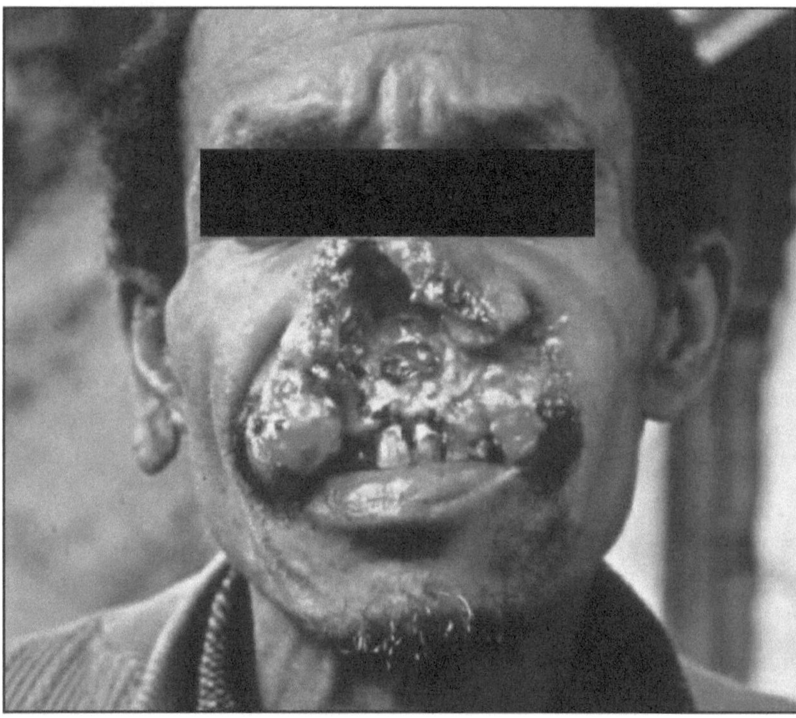

Figure 7: ulcerative-destructive lesion of the mucocutaneous form (photo by P. Desjeux(23))

2.3. Visceral leishmaniasis (LV)

The species responsible for the visceral form of Leishmaniasis *are : L. donovani* and *L. infantum* in the Old World and *L. chagasi* in the New World. Recently, a few cases due to *L. tropica* have also been reported. The population at risk includes pre-school children, the immunocompromised and the undernourished. Lately, it has been observed with increasing frequency in HIV patients. After an incubation period of 3 to 8 months, the course may be subclinical or frankly symptomatic. The clinical picture includes adenopathy, hepatosplenomegaly, pallor, fever, night sweats, weakness, anorexia and weight loss. VL is usually associated with pancytopenia and hypergammaglobulinemia. In adults, the clinical picture is much less typical than in children. A bistre pigmentation of the skin of the face, hands, feet and abdomen is commonly observed in India (the Hindi name of the disease, kala-azar, means "black fever" or "deadly fever"). If left untreated, the disease is fatal (12,15,22).

3. Leishmaniasis in Tunisia

Only two clinical forms have been described in Tunisia: localized cutaneous leishmaniasis and visceral leishmaniasis.

3.1. Cutaneous leishmaniasis

In Tunisia, cutaneous leishmaniasis exists in three forms. These are differentiated by their geographical distribution, their clinical-epidemiological aspect and the species of the causal agent. For a long time, the characterization of these forms was based simply on geographical distribution. However, recent extensions of distribution areas have made it difficult and imprecise to use geographical criteria alone to classify the different forms of cutaneous leishmaniasis in Tunisia(24).

3.1.1. Zoonotic cutaneous leishmaniasis (LCZ)

Epidemiology

Historically, LC in Tunisia was typically sporadic and occasionally epidemic in the Gafsa region at the end of the 19th century, hence the name "Gafsa nail". In 1982, an outbreak of LC occurred near the Sidi Saad dam (Kairouan governorate). In the years that followed, the disease spread to neighboring regions in the west, east and south. Recently, it has spread to the north of the country. This clinical form has been identified as zoonotic, with an annual incidence ranging from 1,000 to 10,000 cases, and occurs in the form of seasonal epidemics. Emerging cases peak in autumn, mainly between September and November(24,25).

Leishmania major is the species responsible for this clinical form. Isoenzymatic characterization showed the presence of a principal zymodeme : MON-25, with wild rodents *Psammomys obesus*, *Meriones shawi* and *Meriones nivalis* as reservoir hosts and *Phlebotomus papatasi* as vector (24,26).

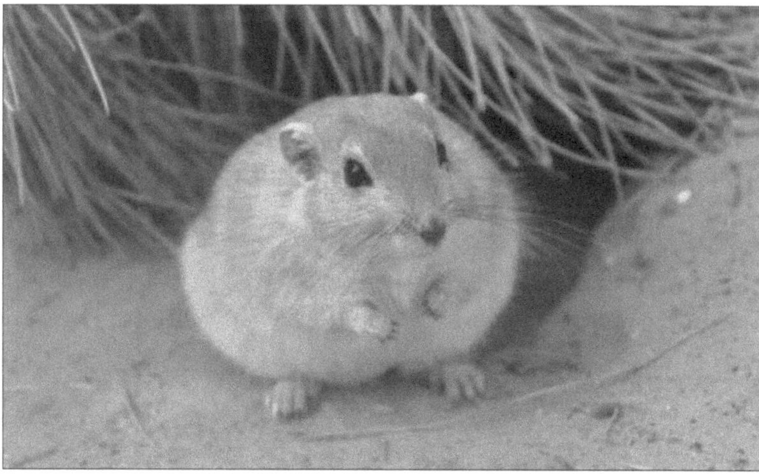

Figure 8: *Psammomys obesus* (27)

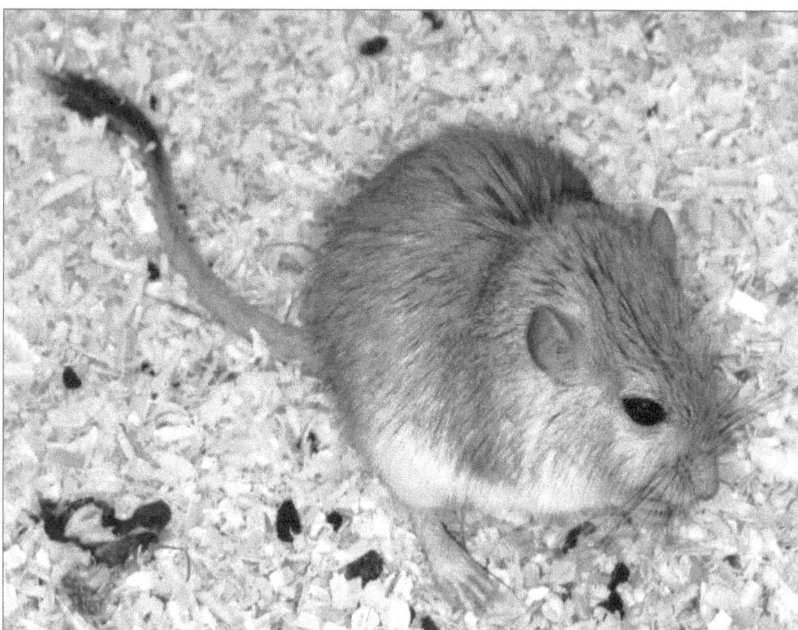

Figure 9: *Meriones shawi* (28)

Clinic

The classic lesion caused by *Leishmania major* is of the "wet" type, with a large central ulceration covered by an adherent crust. LCZ lesions are usually multiple, localized on the limbs and frequently complicated by bacterial superinfections. The incubation period is often less than four months. Recovery is spontaneous in less than 8 months, with residual scarring. A total of twelve different clinical forms of LCZ have been reported. The most common type was ulcerative-crusty, followed by papulonodular and impetiginous. Less common were the ulcerated, mucocutaneous, lupoid and sporotrichoid forms. Eczematiform, erysipeloid, verrucous, psoriasiform and pseudotumoral types were rarer (25,26,29).

3.1.2. Sporadic cutaneous leishmaniasis (SCL)

Epidemiology

The annual incidence of CSF is estimated at 30 cases per year. It is caused by *L. infantum*, whose isoenzymatic characterization has shown the presence of three zymodemes: MON-24 (the most frequent), MON-1 and MON-80. This clinical form, whose reservoir is still unknown, was mainly confined to the north of the country. Recently, a central spread has been reported. Because of its abundance in CSF outbreaks, *Phlebotomus perfiliewi* was thought to be the vector of this disease. However, no *Leishmania infantum (L. infantum)* has been isolated from this species. *Phlebotomus langeroni* and *Phlebotomu longicuspis* are other suspected vectors, as *L. infantum* DNA has been detected in these species(24,26,30).

Clinic

Most patients infected with *L. infantum* present with a single, small, ulcerated or lupoid lesion on the face, surrounded by a large area of infiltration. The evolution of the lesion can last up to three years(26).

3.1.3. Chronic cutaneous leishmaniasis (CCL)

Epidemiology

The pathogen of CCL is *Leishmania killicki (L. killicki),* with two zymodemes: MON-8, the most common, and MON-317, recently identified (26). The taxonomic status of *L. killicki* is not yet well defined (29). This clinical form was first identified in 1980 in the rocky mountains of the Tataouine region. However, since 2005, new outbreaks have emerged in the center and southwest of the country. Annual incidence is estimated at 10 cases per year (31-33).

Until 2011, the transmission cycle was considered anthroponotic. Recently, several studies have confirmed that *Ctenodactylus gundi* (Figure 8) is the reservoir of *L. killicki* in Tunisia, and that *P. sergenti* probably plays the role of vector in the transmission cycle (32,34).

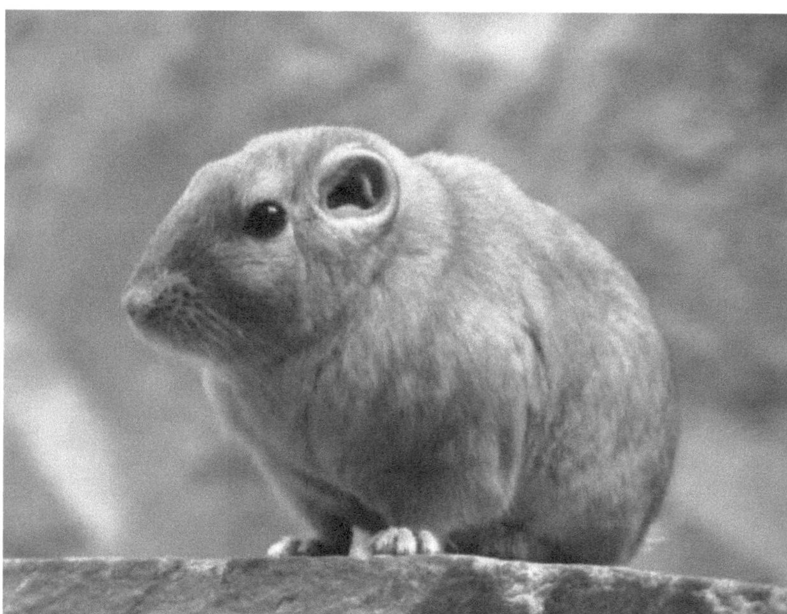

Figure 10: *Ctenodactylus gundi* (35)

Clinic

In LCC, the lesion is single, dry, localized on the face or limbs, and may last up to six years (26).

3.1.4. Visceral leishmaniasis

In Tunisia, the incidence of VL is 100 cases per year. In 95% of cases, it develops in children under the age of five. Initially, it was distributed in the north of the country, notably in Zaghouan, Kef, Jendouba, Seliana, Nabeul, Beja and Tunis. It then spread to the center and south.

As in all countries of the Mediterranean basin, L. infantum is the sole etiological agent of VL in Tunisia. Isoenzymatic analyses have shown that zymodeme MON-1 is the most frequent, followed by MON-24 and MON-80. For MON-1, the transmission cycle is well known, with the domestic dog as the reservoir and *P. perniciosus* as the vector. However, for MON-24 and MON-80, the reservoirs and vectors are still poorly identified (4,24,26,29,36).

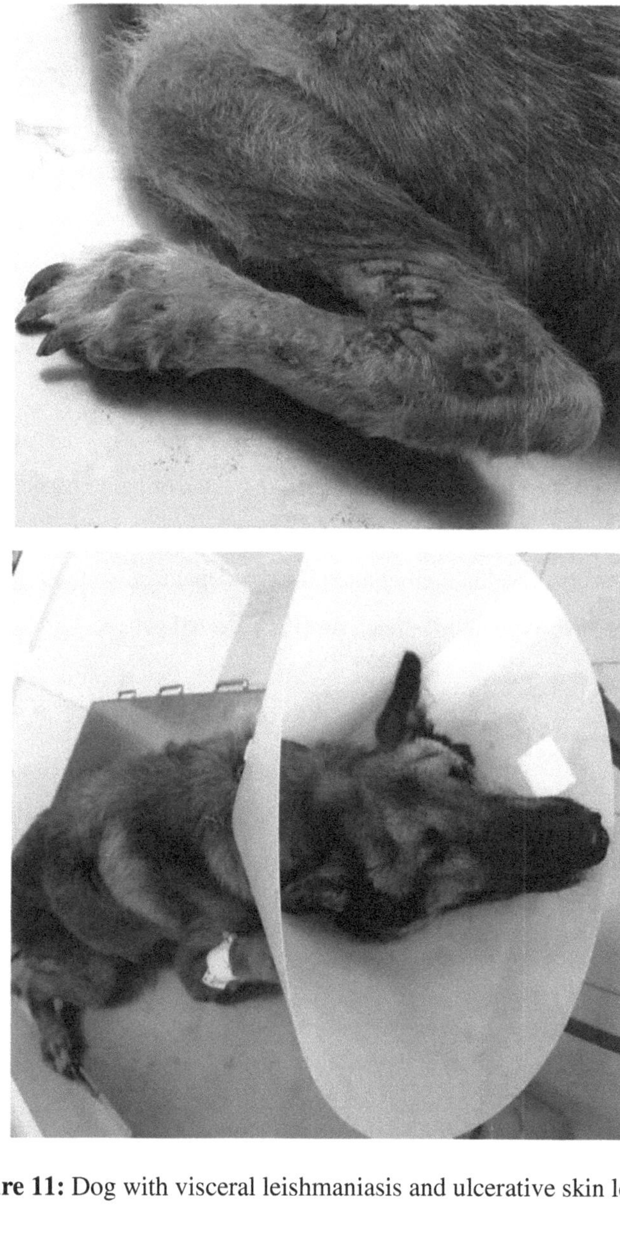

Figure 11: Dog with visceral leishmaniasis and ulcerative skin lesions

4. Diagnosis

Diagnosis of leishmaniasis is based on clinical, epidemiological and biological data. Diagnosis of certainty is provided by detection of the parasite by microscopy, culture or PCR. Immunological diagnosis is reserved for the visceral form (37).

4.1. Microscopic examination

For cutaneous leishmaniasis, amastigotes are detected on samples taken from the inner edge of the lesion. For visceral leishmaniasis, bone marrow aspiration is frequently used, with a sensitivity of around 60% to 85%. Splenic aspiration has a higher sensitivity, but is associated with a high risk of hemorrhage. Leukocyte layer examination has the advantage of being non-invasive, but there are often very few parasitized cells in circulation. Microscopic examination of peripheral blood smears is recommended mainly in HIV-infected patients with VL (18,38).

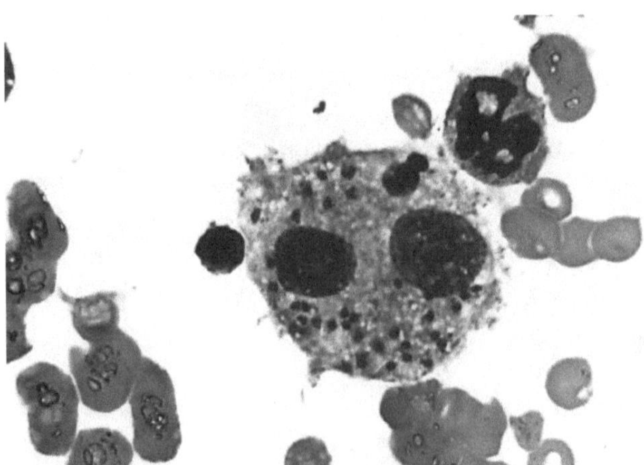

Figure 12: Leishmania body in intracellular position on microscopic examination of a medullary smear.

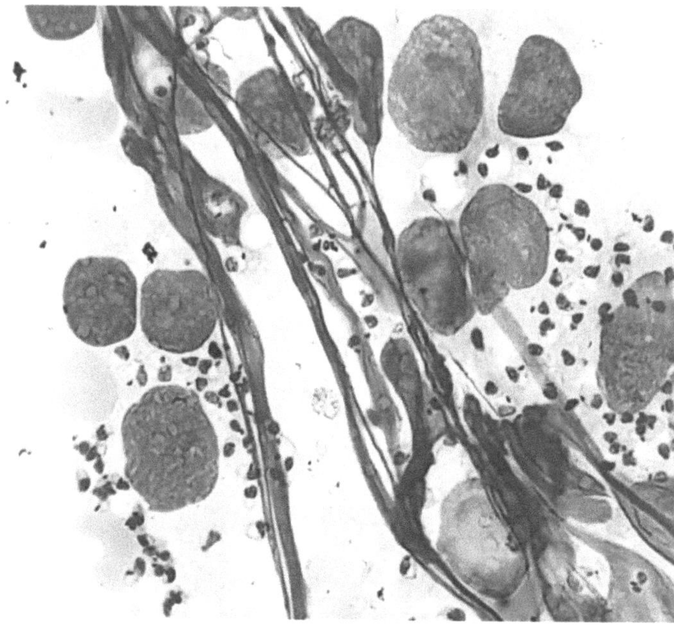

Figure 13: amasigote forms of leishmania in an MGG-stained dermal smear

4.2. Cultivation

Culture of the parasite can improve diagnostic sensitivity. *In vitro,* amastigotes are converted into motile promastigotes. Typically, samples of various types are seeded in culture on Novy Mac-Neal Nicolle (NNN) medium. This is a two-phase medium with a solid phase based on a pellet of salted agar with 10% defibrinated rabbit blood, and a liquid phase consisting of the exudate produced from the blood agar; it is in this liquid phase that the promastigotes develop. The nature and volume of this liquid phase can be supplemented (RPMI medium, fetal calf serum). Incubation takes place at 24-27°C. Verification is carried out once a week, and the culture is not declared negative until the fourth week, after successive subculturing on fresh medium. If positive, mobile flagellate promastigotes are observed under microscopy (Le Fichoux et al, 1999). This technique is limited to research laboratories(18,39,40).

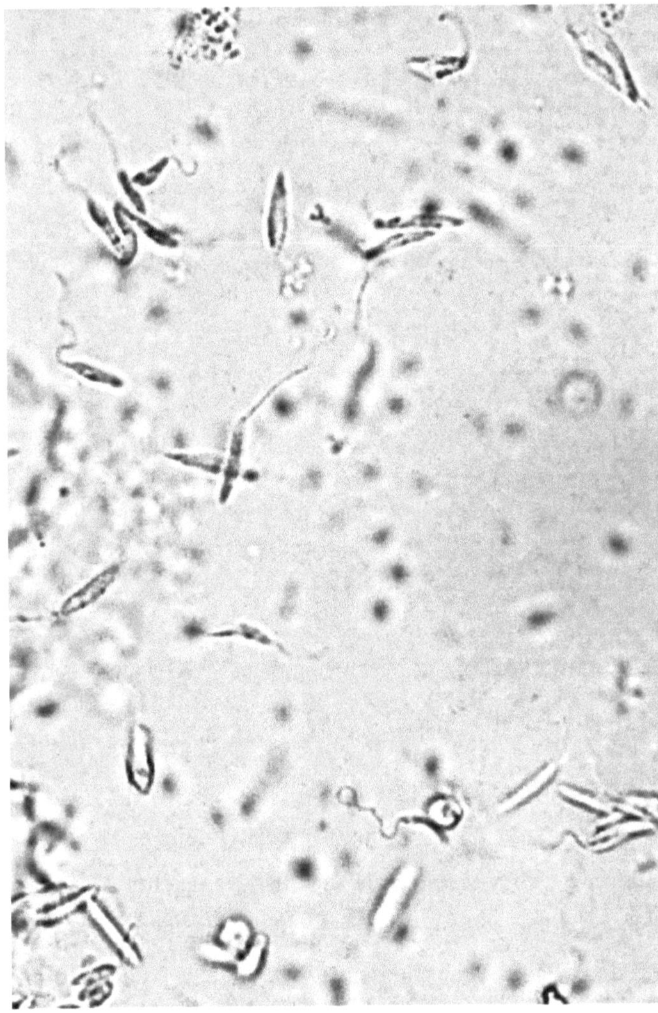

Figure 14: Amastigote form of Leishmania obtained by culture on a medium based on horse blood (Laboratory of Parasitology-Medical and Molecular Mycology, Faculty of Pharmacy, Monastir).

4.3. Immunological diagnosis

Immunological diagnosis is reserved solely for the visceral form of leishmaniasis. It's important to note that a positive serological test is not definitive proof of the presence of active VL. In subjects co-infected with HIV, serological tests have limited diagnostic value: over 40% of these patients have no detectable antibody levels. Serological test results must therefore be interpreted with caution, taking into account clinical, biological and epidemiological information (18). The main serological tests developed are :

Montenegro skin test

The *Leishmania* intradermal skin test or Montenegro skin test is a marker of the cellular immune response, exploiting the delayed-type hypersensitivity reaction. It is based on intradermal injection of a suspension of killed promastigotes. This test is very useful for epidemiological studies, thanks to its simplicity and sensitivity. However, it has very little diagnostic value. Indeed, the test remains negative in active kala-azar, then becomes positive within two months of successful treatment (41).

Direct agglutination test

This test is semi-qualitative. It is widely used in the field. It has been validated in several countries. Its sensitivity ranges from 70.5 to 100%. Specificity ranges from 53 to 100% (37).

Indirect immunofluorescence

For this test, the promastigote form of the parasite, obtained by *in vitro* culture, is used as the antigen source. The test has a sensitivity of 87% to 100% and a specificity of 77% to 100%. It is positive in the early stages of infection and becomes undetectable six to nine months after recovery, making it useful detecting any relapses. The need for a fluorescence microscope limits the use of this test to certain reference laboratories (18).

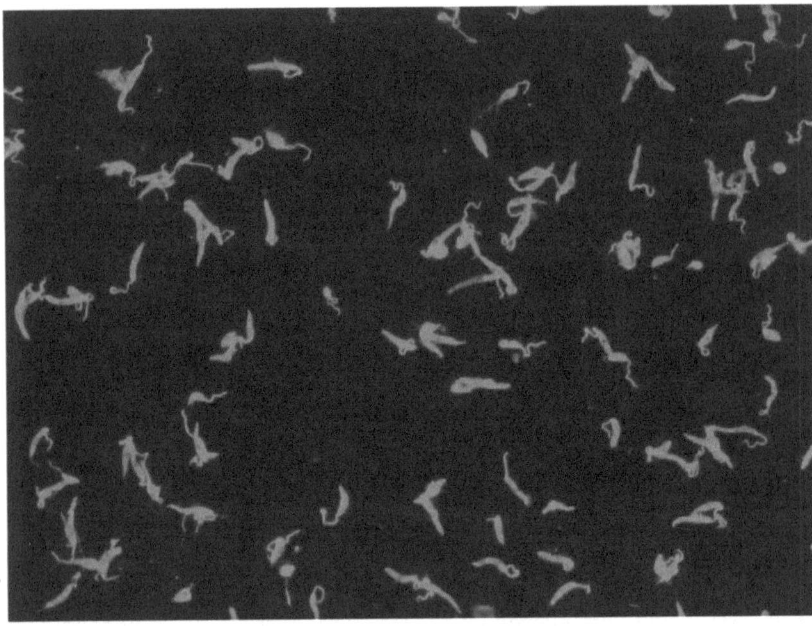

Figure 15: positive indirect immunofluorescence reaction with promastigotes as antigens

ELISA

The sensitivity and specificity of ELISA detection of anti-leishmanial antibodies depend mainly on the nature of the antigen used. In the past, crude parasitic antigens were used, with the common risk of cross-reactivity with other infectious agents. Nowadays, with the advent of technology, several recombinant antigens have been produced, resolving the old problems of lack of specificity (37).

Rapid screening test

This is an immunochromatographic test. It is a qualitative test with the advantages of being reproducible, economical, easy and rapid. The antigen used is the recombinant K39 protein. It offers high sensitivity and specificity in most endemic regions (37).

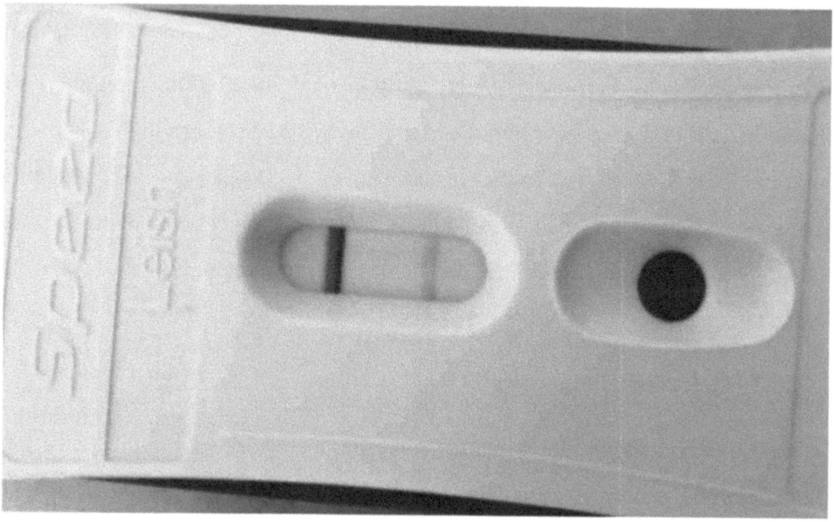

Figure 16: Positive rapid test for visceral leihmaniasis

Western blot

This technique is highly sensitive, making it particularly useful in cases of immunosuppression. However, its high cost limits its use (18).

In addition to antibody testing, parasitic antigens can be tested for in visceral leishmaniasis.

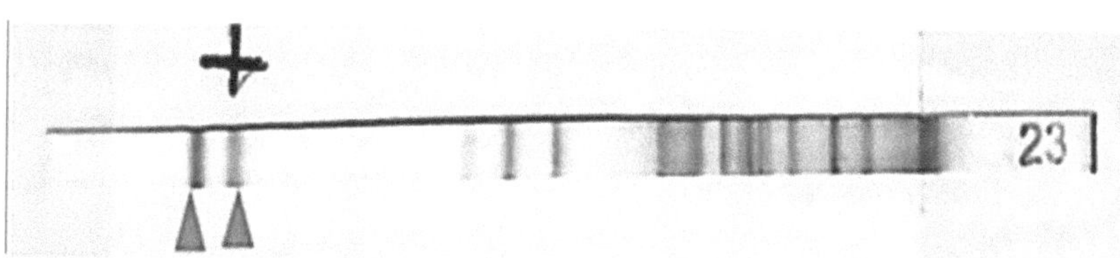

Figure 17: A Western blot of positive leishmaniasis serology showing the presence of the 14 and 16 kDa bands.

Latex agglutination test

This test detects a thermostable glycoprotein of 5 to 20 kDa, present in VL patients, in urine. It's an easy, rapid and non-invasive test. It has high specificity, but low to moderate sensitivity. It has proven its usefulness in therapeutic monitoring, as it rapidly becomes negative following successful treatment. It is also of great interest in cases of deficient antibody production. For example, it can be used to detect VL in HIV patients (42).

4.3.1. Molecular diagnostics

To date, several molecular methods have been developed for the detection, identification, quantification and phylogenetic analysis of leishmaniasis (4,31,43-46).

The sensitivity of these techniques varies according to :

- The nature of the biological sample. For example, in LC, biological material from a biopsy is richer in leishmaniasis than material scraped from the inner edge of the lesion, making PCR more sensitive(47).
- The target tested: the sensitivity of PCR is higher when it is a repeated locus than when it is a single locus in the *Leishmania* genome (48,49). Examples include kinetoplast DNA (1000-10000 mini circles per cell) (50), genes coding for ribosomal RNA and ITS (6 copies on chromosome 27 of the *L. major* genome) (51) and the mini-exon gene (100 to 200 tandemly repeated copies per nuclear genome) (52).

However, the major drawback of this technique is the lack of standardization, mainly due to the use of a wide range of experimental protocols in different laboratories(53).

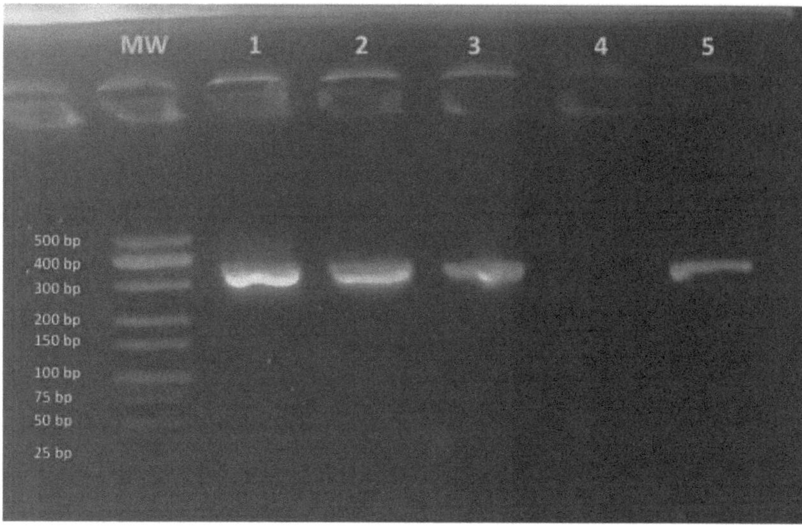

Figure 18: Agarose gel electrophoresis of 18S rRNA PCR product. MW: Molecular weight marker, wells 1, 2 and 3: positive results, well 4: negative control, well 5: positive control.

CONCLUSION

L he epidemiological analysis of leishmaniasis reveals a complex mosaic of factors influencing the transmission and distribution of this parasitic disease. The species of the *Leishmania* genus are remarkably diverse. The sandfly, the main vector, plays a fundamental role in the spread of the disease. Reservoirs, mainly dogs and various rodents, are crucial in maintaining the transmission cycle, affecting the prevalence and epidemiology of leishmaniasis.

The geographical distribution of leishmaniasis, which includes visceral, cutaneous and mucocutaneous forms, is influenced by a combination of environmental, social and biological factors. Tropical and subtropical zones on all five continents are particularly affected, with significant variations between countries. Socio-economic factors, population movements, ecological changes and climatic variations modify epidemiological dynamics. HIV co-infection, which aggravates visceral forms, adds a further dimension to this complexity.

In Tunisia, leishmaniasis manifests itself in two forms: cutaneous and visceral. Cutaneous leishmaniasis presents a range of clinical forms, including zoonotic, sporadic and chronic, each with its own epidemiological and clinical characteristics. In-depth surveillance and targeted research are essential to understand the local dynamics of the parasitosis and adapt control strategies to the particularities of endemic foci.

In conclusion, a global approach integrating the multiple factors influencing the transmission and distribution of leishmaniasis is essential to optimize prevention and treatment strategies. This approach would not only help to better understand the mechanisms of the disease, but also to improve public health interventions.

BIBLIOGRAPHICAL REFERENCES

1. Akhoundi M, Kuhls K, Cannet A, Votypka J, Marty P, Delaunay P, et al. A Historical Overview of the Classification, Evolution, and Dispersion of Leishmania Parasites and Sandflies. PLoS Negl Trop Dis [Internet]. 2016 March 3 [cited 2019 March 29];10(3). Available from:

   https://www.ncbi.nlm.nih.gov/pmc/articles/PMC4777430/

2. Saf'janova VM. Classification of the genus Leishmania Ross. Chapter 11 (in Russian). In: The Leishmaniasis. Protozoology, Academy of Sciences, USSR All Union Society ofProtozoologists, Lennigrad, Part 7, 1982; p. 95-101.

3. Lainson R, Shaw JJ. Evolution, classification and geographical distribution In: Peters W, Killick-Kendrick R editors. The Leishmaniases in Biology and Medicine, Academic Press, London, 1987; p. 1-120.

4. Chargui N, Haouas N, Jaouadi K, Gorcii M, Pratlong F, Dedet JP, et al. Usefulness of a PCR-based method in the detection and species identification of Leishmania from clinical samples. Pathol Biol (Paris). dec 2012;60(6):e75-79.

5. Rioux JA, Lanotte G, Serres E, Pratlong F, Bastien P, Perieres J. Taxonomy of Leishmania. Use of isoenzymes. Suggestions for a new classification. Ann Parasitol Hum Comparée [Internet]. 1990 [cited 8 Apr 2019];65(3):111-25. Available from: https://www.parasite-journal.org/articles/parasite/abs/1990/03/parasite1990653p111/parasite1990653p 111.html

6. Garnham PCC. The genus Leishmania. Bull World Health Organ [Internet]. 1971 [cited 29 March 2019];44(4):477-89. Available from:

   https://www.ncbi.nlm.nih.gov/pmc/articles/PMC2427834/

7. CDC - DPDx - Leishmaniasis [Internet]. 2019 [cited 13 Apr 2019]. Available from: https://www.cdc.gov/dpdx/leishmaniasis/index.html

8. Masson E. Leishmaniasis, leishmanioses. Biology, clinic and therapeutics [Internet]. EM-Consulte. [cited 2019 March 29]. Available from: https://www.em- consulte.com/article/11876/leishmanies-leishmanioses-biology-clinical-and-the

9. Leishrisk, Bridging Research and Leishmanianis Control [Internet]. [cited 13 Apr 2019]. Available from:

http://www.leishrisk.net/leishrisk/Default.aspx?Menu=MenuMain&MIID=34& WPID=40&L=E

10. Akhoundi M, Kuhls K, Cannet A, Votypka J, Marty P, Delaunay P, et al. A Historical Overview of the Classification, Evolution, and Dispersion of Leishmania Parasites and Sandflies. PLoS Negl Trop Dis. March 2016;10(3):e0004349.

11. Maroli M, Feliciangeli MD, Bichaud L, Charrel RN, Gradoni L. Phlebotomine sandflies and the spreading of leishmaniasis and other diseases of public health concern. Med Vet Entomol. June 2013;27(2): 123-47.

12. Leishmaniasis control: report of the WHO expert committee meeting on leishmaniasis control, Geneva, 22 - 26 March 2010 [Internet]. [cited 2019 May 20]. Available from: https://apps.who.int/iris/handle/10665/44634

13. Sacks D, Kamhawi S. Molecular aspects of parasite-vector and vector-host interactions in leishmaniasis. Annu Rev Microbiol. 2001;55:453-83.

14. Harhay MO, Olliaro PL, Costa DL, Costa CHN. Urban parasitology: visceral leishmaniasis in Brazil. Trends Parasitol. 1 Sep 2011;27(9):403-9.

15. WHO | Leishmaniasis [Internet]. WHO. [cited 2019 March 30]. Available from: http://www.who.int/mediacentre/factsheets/fs375/fr/

16. Alemayehu B, Alemayehu M. Leishmaniasis: A Review on Parasite, Vector and Reservoir Host. Health Sci J [Internet]. 2017 Sep 4 [cited 2019 Mar 29];11(4). Available from: http://www.hsj.gr/abstract/leishmaniasis-a-review-on-parasite- vector-and-reservoir-host-20131.html

17. WHO | 10 facts about HIV/AIDS [Internet]. WHO. [cited 20 May 2019]. Available from: http://www.who.int/features/factfiles/hiv/fr/

18. Elmahallawy EK, Sampedro Martinez A, Rodriguez-Granger J, Hoyos-Mallecot Y, Agil A, Navarro Mari JM, et al. Diagnosis of leishmaniasis. J Infect Dev Ctries. August 13, 2014;8(8):961-72.

19. Shafiei R, Mohebali M, Akhoundi B, Galian MS, Kalantar F, Ashkan S, et al. Emergence of co-infection of visceral leishmaniasis in HIV-positive patients in northeast Iran: a preliminary study. Travel Med Infect Dis. Apr 2014;12(2):173-8.

20. Sinha PK, van Griensven J, Pandey K, Kumar N, Verma N, Mahajan R, et al. Liposomal amphotericin B for visceral leishmaniasis in human immunodeficiency virus-coinfected patients: 2-year treatment outcomes in Bihar, India. Clin Infect Dis Off Publ Infect Dis Soc Am. Oct 2011;53(7):e91-98.

21. WHO | Leishmaniasis and HIV coinfection [Internet]. WHO. [cited 2019 May 20]. Available from:

https://www.who.int/leishmaniasis/burden/hiv_coinfection/burden_hiv_coi nfecti on/en/

22. Torres-Guerrero E, Quintanilla-Cedillo MR, Ruiz-Esmenjaud J, Arenas R. Leishmaniasis: a review. F1000Research. 2017;6:750.

23. Course [Internet]. [cited 13 Apr 2019]. Available from: http://campus.cerimes.fr/parasitologie/enseignement/leishmanioses/site/html/4_3 .html

24. Haouas N, Chaker E, Chargui N, Gorcii M, Belhadj S, Kallel K, et al. Geographical distribution updating of Tunisian leishmaniasis foci: about the isoenzymatic analysis of 694 strains. Acta Trop. Dec 2012;124(3):221-8.

25. Aoun K, Bouratbine A. Cutaneous leishmaniasis in North Africa: a review. Parasite Paris Fr. 2014;21:14.

26. Chaara D, Haouas N, Dedet JP, Babba H, Pratlong F. Leishmaniases in Maghreb: an endemic neglected disease. Acta Trop. Apr 2014;132:80-93.

27. Fat sand rat / Psammomys obesus terrasanctae | ZooChat [Internet]. [cited 1 Apr 2019]. Available from: https://www.zoochat.com/community/media/fat-sand-rat- psammomys-obesus-terrasanctae.384760/

28. ondrej.zicha(at)gmail.com OZ. BioLib: Biological library [Internet]. [cited 1 Apr 2019]. Available from: https://www.biolib.cz/en/image/id97965/

29. Haouas N, Babba H. Leishmaniasis in Tunisia: History and New Insights into the Epidemiology of a Neglected Disease. Epidemiol Ecol Leishmaniasis [Internet]. 1 March 2017 [cited 19 May 2019]; Available from:

https://www.intechopen.com/books/the-epidemiology-and-ecology-of-leishmaniasis/leishmaniasis-in-tunisia-history-and-new-insights-into-the-epidemiology-of-a-neglected-disease

30. Chargui N, Slama D, Haouas N, Rmadi L, Babba H. Transmission cycle analysis in a Leishmania infantum focus: Infection rates and blood meal origins in sand flies (Diptera: Psychodidae). J Vector Ecol J Soc Vector Ecol. Dec 2018;43(2):321-7.

31. Haouas N, Chargui N, Chaker E, Ben Said M, Babba H, Belhadj S, et al. Anthroponotic cutaneous leishmaniasis in Tunisia: presence of Leishmania killicki outside its original focus of Tataouine. Trans R Soc Trop Med Hyg. Jul 2005;99(7):499-501.

32. Jaouadi K, Depaquit J, Haouas N, Chaara D, Gorcii M, Chargui N, et al. Twenty-four new human cases of cutaneous leishmaniasis due to Leishmania killicki in Metlaoui, southwestern Tunisia: probable role of Phlebotomus sergenti in the transmission. Acta Trop. June 2012;122(3):276-83.

33. Evolutionary history of Leishmania killicki (synonymous Leishmania tropica) and taxonomic implications. - PubMed - NCBI [Internet]. [cited 22 May 2019]. Available from: https://www.ncbi.nlm.nih.gov/pubmed/25889939

34. Jaouadi K, Haouas N, Chaara D, Gorcii M, Chargui N, Augot D, et al. First detection of Leishmania killicki (Kinetoplastida, Trypanosomatidae) in Ctenodactylus gundi (Rodentia, Ctenodactylidae), a possible reservoir of human cutaneous leishmaniasis in Tunisia. Parasit Vectors. August 11, 2011;4:159.

35. Common Gundi (Ctenodactylus gundi) | ZooChat [Internet]. [cited 1 Apr 2019]. Available from:https://www.zoochat.com/community/media/common-gundi-ctenodactylus-gundi.155554/

36. Besbes A, Pousse H, Ben Said M, Kharrat H, Ghenimi L. Infantile visceral leishmaniasis in central Tunisia (221 cases). Médecine Mal Infect [Internet]. May 1, 1994 [cited 2019 March 30];24(5):628-34. Available on: http://www.sciencedirect.com/science/article/pii/S0399077X05807048

37. Singh OP, Sundar S. Developments in Diagnosis of Visceral Leishmaniasis in the Elimination Era. J Parasitol Res. 2015;2015:239469.

38. Karimi A, Alborzi A, Amanati A. Visceral Leishmaniasis: An Update and Literature Review. Arch Pediatr Infect Dis [Internet]. Jul 1, 2016 [cited 2019 May 20];4(3). Available from: http://pedinfect.com/en/articles/20284.html

39. Le Fichoux Y., Mary C., Marty P., Kubar J. Diagnostic des Leishmanioses. In: Dedet J-P. ed. Les Leishmanioses. Paris, Ellipses; 1999. p. 191-203. In.

40. Cultures on NNN medium in the biological diagnosis of leishmaniasis - EM|consult [Internet]. [cited 22 May 2019]. Available from: https://www.em- consulte.com/en/article/210887

41. Ready PD. Epidemiology of visceral leishmaniasis. Clin Epidemiol. 2014;6:147-54.

42. Elmahallawy EK, Martinez AS, Rodriguez-granger J, Hoyos Y, Agil A, Mari J, et al. Review Article Diagnosis of leishmaniasis. 2014.

43. Spanakos G, Patsoula E, Kremastinou T, Saroglou G, Vakalis N. Development of a PCR-based method for diagnosis of Leishmania in blood samples. Mol Cell Probes. Dec 2002;16(6):415-20.

44. Schonian G, Nasereddin A, Dinse N, Schweynoch C, Schallig HDFH, Presber W, et al. PCR diagnosis and characterization of Leishmania in local and imported clinical samples. Diagn Microbiol Infect Dis. Sept 2003;47(1):349-58.

45. Antinori S, Calattini S, Piolini R, Longhi E, Bestetti G, Cascio A, et al. Is real- time polymerase chain reaction (PCR) more useful than a conventional PCR for the clinical management of leishmaniasis? Am J Trop Med Hyg. Jul 2009;81(1):46-51.

46. Koltas IS, Eroglu F, Uzun S, Alabaz D. A comparative analysis of different molecular targets using PCR for diagnosis of old world leishmaniasis. Exp Parasitol. May 2016;164:43-8.

47. Rotureau B, Ravel C, Couppié P, Pratlong F, Nacher M, Dedet J-P, et al. Use of PCR-Restriction Fragment Length Polymorphism Analysis To Identify the Main New World Leishmania Species and Analyze Their Taxonomic Properties and Polymorphism by Application of the Assay to Clinical Samples. J Clin Microbiol [Internet]. Feb 2006 [cited 6 Apr 2019];44(2):459-67. Available from: https://www.ncbi.nlm.nih.gov/pmc/articles/PMC1392689/

48. Haouas N, Garrab S, Gorcii M, Khorchani H, Chargui N, Ravel C, et al. Development of a polymerase chain reaction-restriction fragment length polymorphism assay for Leishmania major/Leishmania killicki/Leishmania infantum discrimination from clinical samples, application in a Tunisian focus. Diagn Microbiol Infect Dis. Oct 2010;68(2): 152-8.

49. Laurent T, Van der Auwera G, Hide M, Mertens P, Quispe-Tintaya W, Deborggraeve S, et al. Identification of Old World Leishmania spp. by specific polymerase chain reaction amplification of cysteine proteinase B genes and rapid dipstick detection. Diagn Microbiol Infect Dis. Feb 2009;63(2):173-81.

50. Aransay AM, Scoulica E, Tselentis Y. Detection and identification of Leishmania DNA within naturally infected sand flies by seminested PCR on minicircle kinetoplastic DNA. Appl Environ Microbiol. May 2000;66(5):1933-8.

51. Ivens AC, Peacock CS, Worthey EA, Murphy L, Aggarwal G, Berriman M, et al. The genome of the kinetoplastid parasite, Leishmania major. Science. 15 Jul 2005;309(5733):436-42.

52. Marfurt J, Nasereddin A, Niederwieser I, Jaffe CL, Beck H-P, Felger I. Identification and differentiation of Leishmania species in clinical samples by PCR amplification of the miniexon sequence and subsequent restriction fragment length polymorphism analysis. J Clin Microbiol. July 2003;41(7):3147-53.

53. Andreadou M, Liandris E, Kasampalidis IN, Taka S, Antoniou M, Ntais P, et al. Evaluation of the performance of selected in-house and commercially available PCR and real-time PCR assays for the detection of Leishmania DNA in canine clinical samples. Exp Parasitol. August 2012;131(4):419-24.

Kolibri 360 GmbH
Ferdinand-Jühlke-Straße 7
99095 Erfurt, Deutschland
produktsicherheit@kolibri360.de

Druck:
CPI Druckdienstleistungen GmbH
im Auftrag der
Kolibri 360 GmbH
Ferdinand-Jühlke-Str. 7
99095 Erfurt